NATURAL CURE TO HIGH BLOOD PRESSURE

I0454401

15 Natural Ways to Cure Your Blood Pressure

Hudson Sebastian

Table of Contents

CHAPTER I

Description

What Is Blood Pressure?

Blood pressure is the stress of blood pushing in opposition to the partitions of your arteries. Arteries deliver blood from your coronary heart to different parts of your body.

Your blood pressure generally rises and falls all through the day.

What Do Blood Pressure Numbers Imply?

Blood pressure is measured the usage of numbers:

The first wide variety, called systolic blood pressure, measures the pressure in your arteries whilst your heart beats.

The 2d number, known as diastolic blood pressure, measures the pressure in your arteries when your heart rests among beats.

If the size reads a 120 and 80 diastolic, you would say, "one hundred twenty over 80," or write, "one hundred twenty/80 mmHg."

What Are Ordinary Blood Pressure Numbers?

A normal blood pressure level is much less than 120/80 mmHg.1

No count your age, you can take steps every day to hold your blood pressure in a healthy range.

What Do Blood Pressure Numbers Suggest?

Blood pressure is measured the use of numbers:

The first range, referred to as systolic blood pressure, measures the pressure for your arteries whilst your heart beats.

The second quantity, known as diastolic blood pressure, measures the pressure in your arteries while your heart rests among beats.

If the dimension reads 120 systolic and 80 diastolic, you will say, "a hundred and twenty over eighty," or write, "a hundred and twenty/80 mmHg."

What Is Excessive Blood Pressure (High Blood Pressure)?

High blood pressure, additionally called hypertension, is blood pressure this is better than every day. Your blood pressure adjustments at some point of the day based in your activities. Having blood pressure measures constantly above ordinary may additionally bring about an analysis of high blood strain (or high blood pressure).

The better your blood pressure tiers, the more risk you have for different health issues, together with coronary heart disorder, coronary heart assault, and stroke.

Your health care group can diagnose excessive blood pressure and make remedy selections through reviewing your systolic and diastolic blood pressure degrees and comparing them to tiers located in positive guidelines.

The guidelines used to diagnose high blood pressure may additionally differ from health care expert to health care expert:

• Some fitness care professionals diagnose sufferers with excessive blood stress if their blood strain is continuously 140/90 mm Hg or better.2 this limit is based on a guideline launched in 2003, as visible in the table underneath.

• Other fitness care experts diagnose sufferers with high blood stress if their blood pressure is continuously 130/80 mm Hg or better.

What causes high blood pressure?

High blood pressure usually develops over time. It can happen because of unhealthy lifestyle choices, such as not getting enough regular physical activity. Certain health conditions, such as diabetes and having obesity, can also increase the risk for developing high blood pressure. High blood pressure can also happen during pregnancy.

What problems does high blood pressure cause?

High blood pressure can damage your health in many ways. It can seriously hurt important organs like your heart, brain, kidneys, and eyes.

The good news is that, in most cases, you can manage your blood pressure to lower your risk for serious health problems.

CHAPTER II

15 Natural Ways to Treat High Blood Pressure

High blood pressure can harm the heart through the years. Ways of reducing blood pressure consist of regular exercise, weight management, and nutritional modifications.

High blood pressure affects nearly half of American adults and 1 billion humans international.

If left uncontrolled, excessive blood strain increases your danger of coronary heart disease and stroke.

However, there are a range of of things you may do to decrease your blood pressure certainly, even without medicine.

Here Are 15 Natural Ways To Treat High Blood Pressure.

1. Walk and Exercising Often

Share on

Exercise is one of the first-rate matters you may do to decrease high blood stress.

Regular workout helps make your coronary heart more potent and extra efficient at pumping blood, which lowers the strain for your arteries.

In fact, getting a hundred and fifty mins in line with week of moderate exercising, such as walking, or seventy five mins according to week of vigorous exercising, together with running, can assist decrease blood stress and improve coronary heart fitness.

Additionally, a few studies suggests that doing extra exercise than this reduces your blood stress even similarly.

Bottom line: Walking for simply half-hour an afternoon can help decrease your blood pressure.

Getting more exercising enables lessen it even in addition.

2. Reduce Your Sodium Consumption

Salt intake is excessive round the world. This is basically due to improved intake of processed and prepared foods.

Many studies have related high salt intake with high blood pressure and heart occasions, such as stroke.

However, different research shows that the connection among sodium and excessive blood pressure is much less clear.

One cause for this could be genetic variations in how humans process sodium. About half of people with high blood strain and 1 / 4 of people with normal stages seem to have a sensitivity to salt. If you already have high blood pressure, it's worth cutting returned your sodium consumption to see whether or not it makes a distinction. Swap processed foods for clean elements and strive seasoning with herbs and spices as opposed to salt.

Bottom line: Most hints for lowering blood stress propose reducing sodium consumption.

However, that advice would possibly make the maximum experience for folks who are sensitive to the results of salt.

3. Drink Much Less Alcohol

Drinking alcohol can improve blood pressure and boom the danger of several continual health conditions, such as high blood strain.

While some research has suggested that low to moderate quantities of alcohol consumption might also guard the coronary heart, the ones benefits may be offset by negative effects.

In the United States, moderate alcohol consumption is described as no a couple of drink according to day for females and drinks per day for men. If you drink greater than that, it might be quality to do not forget reducing your intake.

Bottom line: Drinking any amount of alcohol might also enhance your blood pressure. Therefore, it's quality to mild your consumption.

4. Eat Extra Potassium-Rich Meals

Potassium is a crucial mineral that facilitates your frame dispose of sodium and eases stress on your blood vessels.

Modern diets have multiplied most human being's sodium consumption whilst lowering potassium intake.

To get a higher balance of potassium and sodium on your food plan, attention on eating fewer processed foods and more sparkling, complete foods.

Foods which might be mainly high in potassium include:

•   Vegetables, especially leafy greens, tomatoes, potatoes, and sweet potatoes

- Fruit, together with melons, bananas, avocados, oranges, and apricots

- Dairy, including milk and yogurt

- Tuna and salmon

- Nuts and seeds

- Beans

Bottom line: Eating clean end result and greens, which can be rich in potassium, can help decrease blood pressure.

5. Cut Back On Caffeine

If you've ever downed a cup of coffee before you've had your blood pressure taken, you'll realize that caffeine reasons an instantaneous blood pressure enhance.

However, there's not a good deal evidence to suggest that ingesting caffeine often can motive a long-lasting boom.

In reality, folks who drink caffeinated espresso or tea tend to have a lower hazard of coronary heart disorder, inclusive of excessive blood pressure, than those who do now not drink it.

Still, if you suspect you're sensitive to the outcomes of caffeine, don't forget cutting again to see whether or not it lowers your blood pressure.

Bottom line: Caffeine can reason a short-time period spike in blood pressure. However, for many people, it does no longer reason an enduring increase.

6. Learn To Manage Stress

Stress is a key motive force of high blood pressure.

When you're chronically stressed, your body is in a regular combat-or-flight mode. On a physical degree, meaning a quicker coronary heart charge and constricted blood vessels.

When you revel in pressure, you may additionally be much more likely to engage in behavior that can have bad effects on blood pressure, inclusive of ingesting alcohol and eating processed ingredients.

Several research have explored how decreasing pressure can help decrease blood pressure. Here are two proof-based totally tips to try:

• Listen to soothing music: Calming track can assist relax your fearful machine. Research has shown that it's an effective complement to other blood stress treatment options.

• Work much less: Working lots and demanding work conditions are each related to excessive blood strain.

Bottom line: Chronic stress can make contributions to excessive blood strain. Finding methods to manage stress can help.

7. Eat Darkish Chocolate Or Cocoa

While eating massive amounts of dark chocolate possibly received help your heart, small quantities can also.

That's because dark chocolate and cocoa powder are wealthy in flavonoids, which can be plant compounds that cause blood vessels to dilate.

A 2017 review of studies discovered that flavonoid-wealthy cocoa might also lessen short-time period blood pressure tiers in wholesome adults.

For the strongest consequences, use non-alkalized cocoa powder, that is in particular excessive in flavonoids and has no delivered sugars.

Bottom line: Dark chocolate and cocoa powder contain plant compounds that help loosen up blood vessels, which may decrease blood pressure.

8. Try to Shed Pounds, If Important

In those who are obese, dropping weight can make a massive difference to coronary heart fitness.

According to a 2016 have a look at, losing five% of your frame weight may want to appreciably decrease excessive blood stress.

The effect is even greater while weight loss is paired with workout.

Losing weight can help your blood vessels do a higher task of expanding and contracting, making it less complicated for the left ventricle of your coronary heart to pump blood.

Bottom line: Losing weight can considerably decrease excessive blood pressure. This impact is even more suggested when you exercise.

9. If You Smoke, Take Into Account Quitting

Among the many reasons to quit smoking is that the addiction is a strong hazard component for heart disease.

Every puff of cigarette smoke reasons a mild, temporary increase in blood strain. The chemical compounds in tobacco also are acknowledged to damage blood vessels.

However, studies haven't observed a conclusive link among smoking and high blood strain. This can be due to the fact folks that smoke often develop a tolerance over time.

Still, considering that both smoking and high blood pressure increase the risk of coronary heart ailment, quitting smoking can assist lessen that danger.

Bottom line: Though there's conflicting research about smoking and excessive blood strain, both boom the chance of heart ailment.

10. Cut Introduced Sugar and Delicate Carbs

There's a developing frame of studies showing a link between brought sugar consumption and high blood strain.

A 2020 research review discovered that accelerated intake of sugar-sweetened liquids become connected to better blood strain tiers in youngsters and young people.

And it's not simply sugar — all delicate carbs, which include the kind determined in white flour, convert rapidly to sugar in your bloodstream and will purpose problems.

Some research have shown that low carb diets may additionally help reduce blood pressure.

In truth, one evaluate of 12 studies showed that following a low carb food regimen should reduce systolic and diastolic blood pressure, alongside numerous other hazard elements for heart disease.

Bottom line: Consuming delicate carbs, specifically sugar, may enhance blood pressure. Some research have shown that low carb diets may additionally help decrease your blood strain levels.

11. Eat Berries

Berries are full of greater than just juicy taste.

They're also filled with polyphenols, natural plant compounds that are correct to your coronary heart.

Polyphenols can reduce the chance of stroke, coronary heart situations, and diabetes and improve blood stress, insulin resistance, and systemic infection.

In one look at, researchers assigned human beings with excessive blood pressure to a low polyphenol food regimen or a high polyphenol diet containing berries, chocolate, fruits, and veggies.

Those ingesting berries and polyphenol-rich ingredients experienced progressed markers of coronary heart sickness danger.

Bottom line: Berries are wealthy in polyphenols that could help lower blood strain and the overall danger of coronary heart ailment.

12. Try Meditation or Deep Breathing

While those behaviors may also fall under "pressure discount strategies," meditation and deep breathing deserve particular mention.

Both meditation and deep respiration may spark off the parasympathetic worried machine. This machine is engaged while the body relaxes, slowing the coronary heart price and reducing blood strain.

There's quite a chunk of research in this area, with research displaying that distinctive styles of meditation appear to have advantages for reducing blood strain.

Deep respiratory strategies also can be pretty powerful.

Practicing diaphragmatic respiratory, a deep respiration technique, twice each day for four weeks should lead to a discount in systolic and diastolic blood pressure.

Bottom line: Both meditation and deep respiration can set off the parasympathetic anxious device, which facilitates slow your coronary heart fee and decrease blood pressure.

13. Eat Calcium-Rich Ingredients

People with low calcium intake regularly have excessive blood pressure.

While calcium dietary supplements haven't been conclusively proven to lower blood strain, calcium-wealthy diets do seem to be related to healthy blood pressure ranges.

For maximum adults, the calcium advice is 1,000 milligrams (mg) according to day. However, a few humans, consisting of older adults, might also need extra.

In addition to dairy, you can get calcium from collard greens and different leafy greens, beans, sardines, and tofu. Here is a list of calcium-wealthy plant-based totally ingredients.

Bottom line: Calcium-wealthy diets are related to wholesome blood stress tiers. You can get calcium by way of ingesting darkish leafy veggies, tofu, and dairy products.

14. Take Herbal Supplements

Some herbal dietary supplements may assist lower blood strain. Here are some of the principle supplements which have proof in the back of them:

- Aged garlic extract: Researchers have used aged garlic extract efficiently as a stand-by myself remedy and at the side of traditional healing procedures for decreasing blood stress.

- Berberine: Though greater studies is wanted, a few research have determined that berberine may want to potentially help lower blood pressure degrees.

- Whey protein: In a 2016 study with 38 members, people who ate up whey protein experienced stepped forward blood strain and blood vessel feature.

- Fish oil: Long credited with improving heart health, fish oil may benefit human beings with excessive blood pressure the most.

- Hibiscus: Hibiscus flowers make a delectable tea. They're rich in anthocyanins and polyphenols that are desirable in your coronary heart and might decrease blood pressure.

Read more about dietary supplements for high blood strain.

Bottom line: Researchers have investigated several herbal dietary supplements for their potential to lower blood stress.

15. Eat Meals Rich in Magnesium

Magnesium is an essential mineral that enables blood vessels loosen up.

While magnesium deficiency is quite rare, many people don't get enough magnesium of their diet.

Some research have advised that obtaining too little magnesium is related with high blood stress, however proof from medical research has been much less clean.

Still, you could make sure which you're assembly your needs by way of enjoying quite a few magnesium-rich foods, along with veggies, dairy merchandise, legumes, chook, pork, and complete grains.

Bottom line: Magnesium is a critical mineral that allows regulate blood stress. It may be discovered in a extensive range of whole ingredients, such as legumes and whole grains.

THE END